Paleo Cookies
Over 30 Healthy & Delicious Gluten Free
Cookies Dessert Recipes

By: *Emily Simmons*

EMILY SIMMONS

PALEO COOKIES, OVER 30 HEALTHY & DELICIOUS GLUTEN FREE COOKIES DESSERT RECIPES

<u>Disclaimer</u>:

Introduction

When we say "Paleo diet", we are referring to following a diet chart which uses ingredients from the Stone Age. But there was not a trace of sugar or dessert in that age. Our ancestors did not even know about it. But what are we to do when we see so many delicious desserts all around us? Our sweet tooth starts craving sweets even more when we look at or smell delicious sweets and foods. However, no need to worry. Even in the Paleo diet, we have a lot of options to make and bake cookies, cakes and desserts using healthy ingredients.

Gluten Free Paleo Cookies offers numerous options for making cookies and other desserts. If you are a chocolate fan, you will find the initial few recipes filled with dark chocolate and cacao. However, if you want a change from chocolate, you can switch to blueberries, lemon, maple syrup, bacon and many other things to satiate your taste buds. You seem to never get enough of unhealthy desserts, but are constantly left craving more. But Paleo desserts are fully satisfying. They satisfy your sweet tooth in the best possible way and do not make you crave sweetness all day long. Moreover, you can indulge in these sweets as much as you want without any guilt because they are made up of absolutely natural ingredients.

People these days are more concerned about their health than ever before. Thus, they prefer remaining hungry to eating unhealthily. But it is neither good for the body nor practical to go without desserts when all your friends are savoring delicacies of cakes and pastries after a dinner. Thus, it has become more of a necessity to have healthy options for main courses as well as

PALEO COOKIES, OVER 30 HEALTHY & DELICIOUS GLUTEN FREE COOKIES DESSERT RECIPES

desserts; not only to satisfy your cravings, but also to maintain your social life.

Open this book and explore a world of beautiful, healthy cookies. Enjoy!

How to Handle your Sweet Tooth Cravings.

It is really next to impossible to escape your cravings for sweet treats. However, we do not mean to discourage you- not at all. Even when you cut down on the usual culprits- candy, simple carbohydrates and desserts, there are many places where sugar can sneak into your diet. Even the healthiest of foods contain a lot of sugar. For instance, 8 ounces of a regular smoothie contains 28 grams of sugar. This is very close to the 26 grams of sugar in a similar quantity of cola. Amazed, aren't you?

Don't worry. We all get cravings for one thing or the other every now and then. Not cheating on your Paleo diet requires a huge amount of will-power and most of us, of course, do not have it. The solution is to know how and where to cheat. When we know the right substitutes, we can cheat the cheating as well!

PALEO COOKIES, OVER 30 HEALTHY & DELICIOUS GLUTEN FREE COOKIES DESSERT RECIPES

Change what cheating means to you

The best way to reduce the effects of cheating is to change the definition of cheating for you. It means that you have to find out about healthier cheat foods for when you have cravings. When you consume these healthier "cheat foods", you can get "off the menu" and still remain healthy.

List your favorite sweet foods from your previous lifestyle. Typically, they are some of these: Nutella, Red Bull, Snickers, peanut butter, ice-creams, doughnuts, etc. Now, you just have to substitute these foods with Paleo alternatives like: dark chocolate, bacon, avocado, raspberries, banana, whipped cream coffee, whipped cream with berries, frozen fruit smoothies, red wine, and almonds.

The most important benefit of these Paleo cheat foods is that most of these are self-limiting foods. You may recall that you could not stop yourself from eating a whole box of vanilla sundae. But you cannot eat a complete bar of very dark chocolate or cacao. You feel satiated early, and when you consume less, you are also consuming fewer calories.

<u>What You Can do to Control Yourself From Eating Non-Paleo Desserts</u>

Everyone needs a break from all those "healthy" foods. You might want to allow yourself to deviate from that healthy path now and again. But no one wants to go back 4 weeks just because of a single craving. Go through the following tips to readjust your cravings.

If there is cheat food in your home, you will eat it

Avoid buying foods that you don't want to eat yourself. Buying ice-cream for the guests who are due to come next week is just an excuse. You know in your heart that you are going to eat it in the next two days. Do not buy it before you need it.

Eat cheat foods that satisfy your cravings

When you eat ice-cream, you feel guilty and unsatisfied afterwards. So, what is the use of eating any such food which does not satisfy your cravings? Instead, eat foods which will satisfy you and not make you feel terrible afterwards.

Think of the prize of being on Paleo

When you remember your goal of a better physique, better moods and good health, you will not feel guilty or deprived while you are on a Paleo diet. If you constantly think of foods that you cannot eat, you will feel negative and more vulnerable to give into temptations of unhealthy foods. If you think positively about the abundance of foods that you *can* eat, you will not feel deprived.

PALEO COOKIES, OVER 30 HEALTHY & DELICIOUS GLUTEN FREE COOKIES DESSERT RECIPES

How to Beat Your Cravings Without Willpower

Controlling your cravings needs much more than just willpower. You can save the willpower for emergency situations, when you just have to control your cravings. Use these methods to tackle your cravings on a day-to-day basis:

You must prevent your cravings

You might be wondering how that's possible. You must eat when you feel hungry. If your stomach calls for food, it's hunger, not craving. Feed your body with quality protein and fat. You will not have as many cravings if your stomach is satisfied. Do not deprive yourself of carbohydrates and fats. When you do, you crave them even more. Eat Paleo friendly carbs and fats.

Distract yourself

You can distract yourself if you feel the craving for anything unhealthy. Try these methods:

Read a novel.

Watch your favorite show on TV.

Open an album of old photos.

Do yoga.

Paint, knit, crochet, sew or do anything to keep yourself busy.

Take a siesta.

Stay happy

You might just be feeling down and thinking of it as cravings. You can do something else to cheer yourself up instead of eating fast food. Try these ideas:

Visit an interesting place.

Take time out just for yourself, even if it is very unproductive. You do not have to answer to anyone for taking a break.

Surprise a friend by randomly showing up.

Do anything that you think is fun.

Do not feel embarrassed about the craving.

Do not let the craving make you feel guilty forever. If you think of it as just a passing phase which everyone experiences, it will become more manageable. Acknowledge it and let it pass.

Replace your cravings

PALEO COOKIES, OVER 30 HEALTHY & DELICIOUS GLUTEN FREE COOKIES DESSERT RECIPES

We have already spoken about this. You can substitute your cheat foods with healthier Paleo foods such as Paleo crackers, Paleo cakes, Paleo cookies, Paleo pizza, Paleo ice-cream etc.

Go to a healthy place

It becomes easier to stop craving pizza if you are not forced to smell it. You get the point, right? Remove yourself physically from the place where you feel more cravings, instead of staying there and trying to fight them.

Paleo Cookies Recipes

Paleo Samoas

These Paleo samoas are just awesome. Serve them chilled and your family will ask for them over and over again.

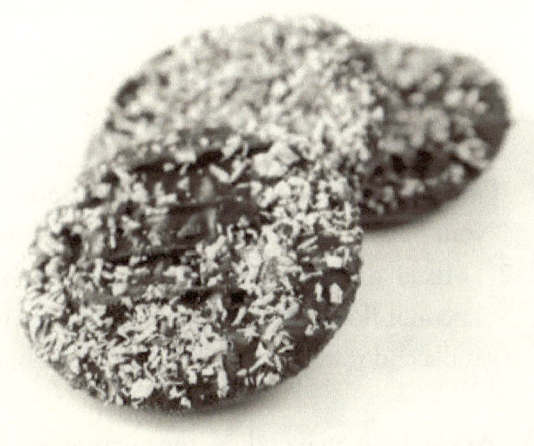

SERVES: 5-6
PREPARATION TIME: 1 hour
INGREDIENTS:
Shortbread cookies:
Almond flour 2 cups
Coconut flour ¼ cup
Coconut sugar ¼ cup
Butter (at room temperature) 10 tablespoons
Vanilla extract 2 teaspoons
Baking soda ¼ teaspoons

Honey caramel:
Raw honey ½ cup
Nut butter (unsalted- cashew, pecan or almond) 2 tablespoons
Vanilla extract 1 teaspoon
Chocolate drizzle:
Chopped cacao butter ½ cup
Cacao powder 5 tablespoons
Raw honey 2 tablespoons
Unsweetened coconut flakes ¼ cup
METHOD (for cookies):

1. Preheat the oven to a temperature of 350 degrees. Line your baking dish with unbleached parchment paper.
2. Mix all dry ingredients for cookies- almond flour, coconut flour, coconut sugar and baking soda. Add vanilla and softened butter. Blend in the butter using a fork.
3. As you keep on blending, the mixture will form into a ball of dough. Wrap it in parchment paper. Refrigerate it for 1 hour.
4. Place the refrigerated dough between two sheets of unbleached parchment paper.
5. Roll it into ¼- ½ inch thick layer.
6. Take a 2.5 inch cookie cutter, and cut out cookies. Roll the dough again and repeat the procedure until you finish the dough.
7. Place the cookies on the baking dish and cook for 12 minutes in the oven or until they become golden brown.
8. Remove the cookies onto a cooling rack. Let cool

PALEO COOKIES, OVER 30 HEALTHY & DELICIOUS GLUTEN FREE COOKIES DESSERT RECIPES

completely.

1.

METHOD (for chocolate drizzle and honey caramel):

1.   Heat a small saucepan over medium heat and add honey. Let it heat for 3-5 minutes and keep stirring occasionally. When you see small bubbles rising from the pan, lower the heat.
2.   Take it off the heat and mix in vanilla and nut butter. The caramel will be in a liquid state when you mix the ingredients and will firm up gradually while cooling down.
3.   Heat another small saucepan over low heat. Melt honey, cacao powder and cacao butter. Cook for 3-5 minutes or until a smooth paste is made. Keep aside.

METHOD (for assembling cookies):

1.   Place the cookies on the baking sheet lined with parchment paper and frost them with caramel. Drizzle chocolate on top of the cookies and sprinkle with coconut flakes.
2.   Refrigerate the cookies and serve chilled.

PALEO COOKIES, OVER 30 HEALTHY & DELICIOUS GLUTEN FREE COOKIES DESSERT RECIPES

1.
2.

<u>Bacon Maple Chocolate Cookies</u>

Bacon never fails to please in the Paleo diet. Apart from being added to other gluten free recipes, bacon pieces taste wonderful in these chocolate cookies as well.

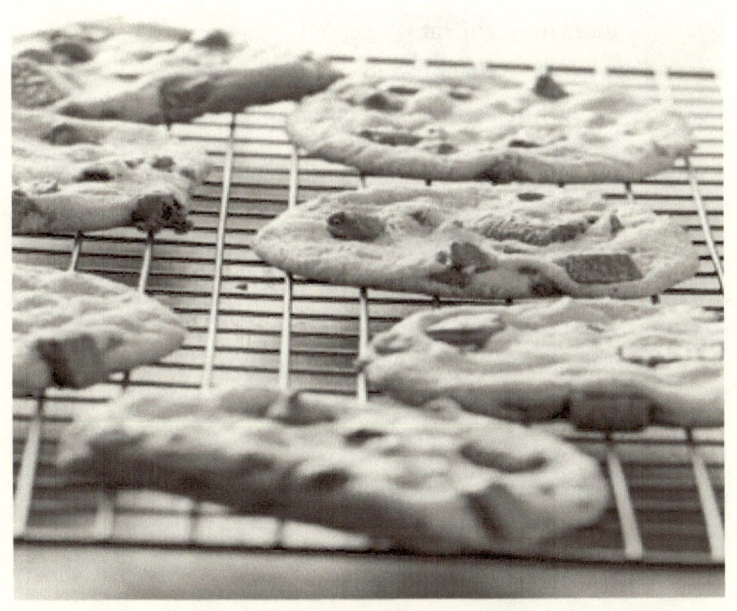

SERVES: 5-6
PREPARATION TIME: 1 hour
INGREDIENTS:
Bacon 4 slices
Bacon fat 2-3 tablespoons
Almond flour 1 cup
Chocolate chips ½ cup

Eggs 2
Maple syrup 3 tablespoons
Vanilla extract 1 teaspoon
METHOD:

1. Preheat the oven to a temperature of 350 degrees Fahrenheit.
2. Take a pan and heat it over medium heat. Cook bacon slices until the fat is released. You can cook some extra slices too for munching on later.
3. While the bacon is cooking, combine all other ingredients (except bacon fat and bacon) and mix properly.
4. When the slices of bacon are cooked, chop them into pieces of ¼– ½ inches. Slightly larger pieces give a better texture to the cookies. Break the pieces using clean hands only.
5.
6. Add the pieces of bacon into the bowl containing other ingredients and add bacon fat. Combine well.
7. Line a baking sheet with aluminum foil and scoop out the mixture in equal measures over the baking sheet. You can use a measuring spoon for this purpose.
8. Put it into the oven and cook for 10 minutes or until you see that the edges have become golden brown. The center will become firm when thoroughly cooked.
9. Serve hot or cooled, as you prefer.

Chocolate Chip Blueberry Cookies

Blueberries have tremendous health benefits. They not only keep your bones healthy, but also help in digestion and to fight wrinkles. So, all the pretty ladies out there! Gobble down these healthy Paleo blueberry cookies without any guilt and reap the benefits.

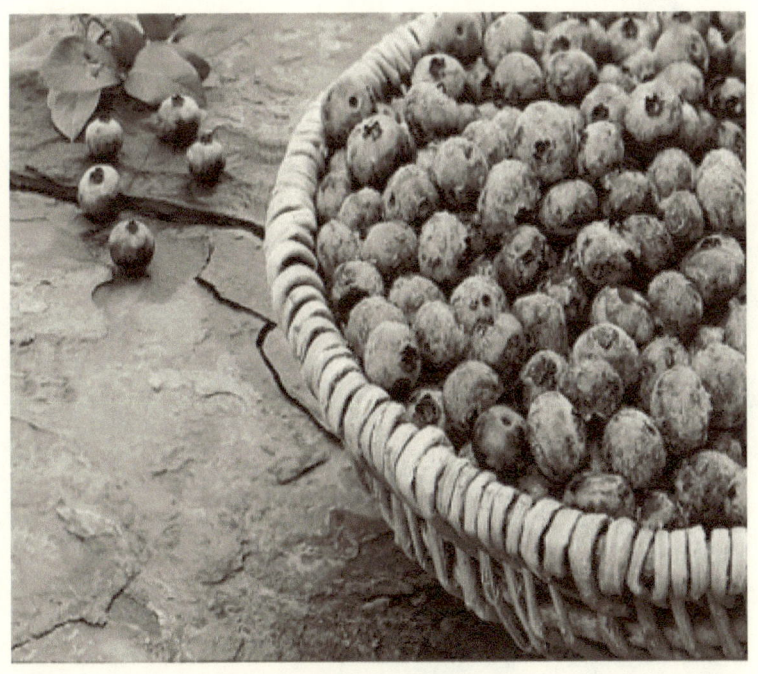

SERVES: 3-4
PREPARATION TIME: 35 minutes
INGREDIENTS:
Blueberries 2 cups
Walnuts 2 cups

EMILY SIMMONS

Walnut oil/ almond oil/ coconut oil 2 tablespoons
Almond flour 1.5 cup
Chocolate chips (dark) 1/3 cup
Maple syrup 3 tablespoons
Whisked egg 1 medium
Cinnamon 1 tablespoon
Vanilla extract 1 teaspoon
Baking soda ¼ teaspoon
Salt a pinch
Coconut crystals for topping

PALEO COOKIES, OVER 30 HEALTHY & DELICIOUS GLUTEN FREE COOKIES DESSERT RECIPES

METHOD:

1. Preheat the oven to a temperature of 400 degrees Fahrenheit.
2. Take a baking sheet and line it with parchment paper.
3. Take a medium saucepan and put blueberries in it over low-medium heat. Let them cook for 10 minutes. Keep stirring frequently.
4. While the blueberries are cooking, add walnuts to the jar of a food processor. Process until the walnuts turn into chunky butter.
5. Now, add blueberries to the jar with walnut butter. Process to blend them together.
6. Take out the batter and place in a large bowl. Put in the rest of the ingredients. Combine them well.
7. Using an ice-cream scoop or a tablespoon, take out 2 scoops of batter for each cookie on the baking sheet. Your batter should make 14-15 cookies.
8. Put the baking tray in the oven and bake for 20-23 minutes.
9. Take the cookies out of the oven and let cool. The cookies may be sticky. If so, use a plastic spatula to remove them when they cool down.
10. Serve.

Chocolate Chip Sweet Potato Cookies

Enjoy your sweet potato cookies with a cup of coffee and indulge in the heavenly taste of these unforgettable cookies.

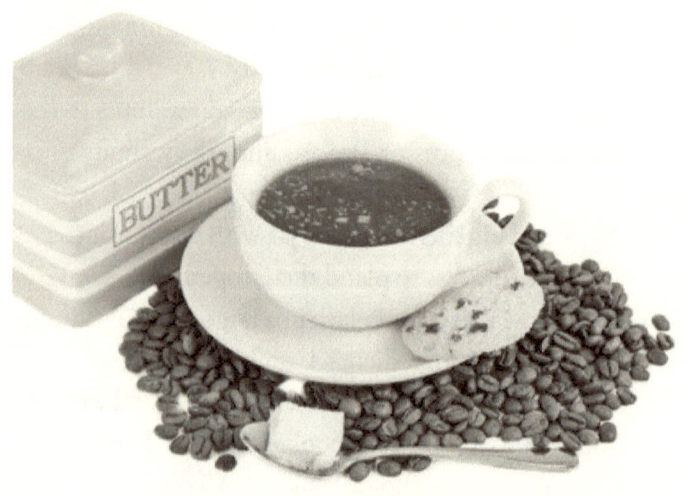

SERVES: 3-4
PREPARATION TIME: 50 minutes
INGREDIENTS:
Sweet potato 1 small
Almond butter (smooth) ½ cup
Whisked egg 1 medium
Honey 1 tablespoon
Vanilla extract 1 teaspoon
Vanilla protein powder 35 grams (1 scoop)
Cinnamon 1/8 teaspoon
Salt a pinch

Chocolate chips ½ cup
METHOD:

1. Preheat the oven to a temperature of 400 degrees Fahrenheit.
2. Poke holes in the potato and place it in the oven to be baked for 35-40 minutes. The potato should become completely soft.
3. Take the potato out and let it cool. Reduce the oven temperature to 350 degrees.
4. Peel the potato and put it in a bowl. Mash it using a fork.
5. Add egg, almond butter, vanilla extract and honey. Combine the ingredients well.
6. Add cinnamon powder, salt, and protein powder to the same bowl. Mix them well.
7. Add chocolate chips and fold them in well.
8. Take a baking sheet and line it with parchment paper.
9. Take tablespoons of the batter and place them on the baking sheet. 12-13 cookies can be made with this amount of batter.
10. Place the baking sheet in the oven and cook for 10-12 minutes. Take out the cookies and let cool. Serve. You can also sprinkle some chocolate chips on top of the cookies immediately after you take them out of the oven.

Chocolate Chunk Cookies

Very easy to make and quick to cook- these cookies are just the thing when your sweet tooth wants something urgently! Cook them in a jiffy and enjoy!

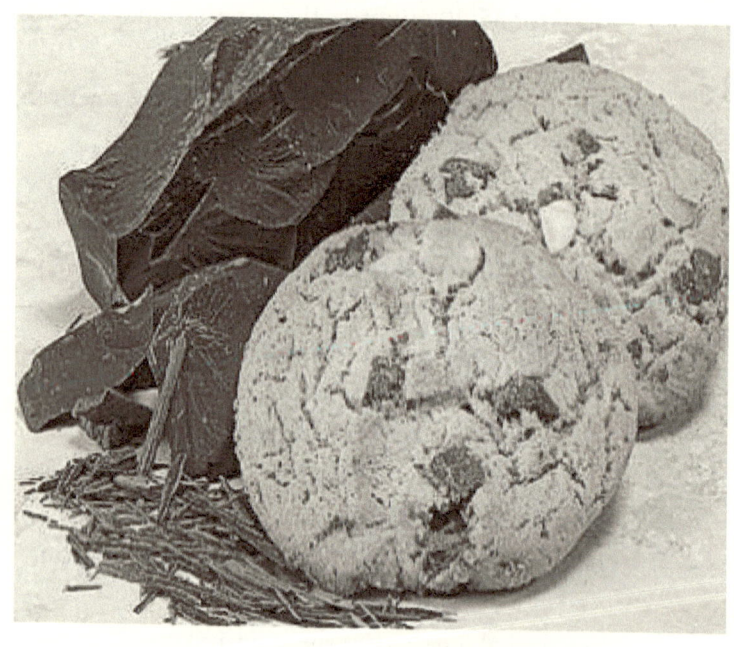

SERVES: 3
PREPARATION TIME: 20 minutes
INGREDIENTS:
Sunflower seed butter (chunky) 1 cup
Honey 1/3 cup
Egg 1
Vanilla 1 teaspoon
Cinnamon 1 tablespoon

PALEO COOKIES, OVER 30 HEALTHY & DELICIOUS GLUTEN FREE COOKIES DESSERT RECIPES

Baking powder ½ teaspoon
Baking soda ½ teaspoon
Salt as per taste
Chopped walnuts ½ cup
Chocolate chunks ½ cup

METHOD:

1. Preheat the oven to a temperature of 350 degrees Fahrenheit.
2. Take a medium sized bowl and put in all the ingredients. Mix well.
3. Take a baking dish and line it with parchment paper.
4. Take a large spoon put scoops of the batter onto the baking dish. Leave plenty of space between each scoop.
5. Put the dish into the preheated oven and cook for 12-15 minutes.
6. Take the dish out and serve cookies.

Chocolate Cranberry Cookies

Again, you have a recipe that's easy to make and just delicious.
Cranberry cookies. They look lovely, and they taste amazing as
well.

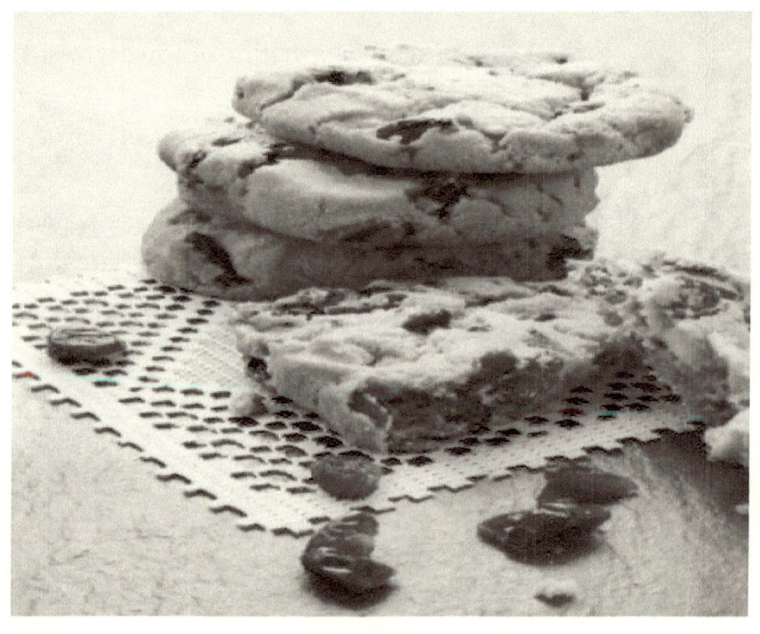

SERVES: 4
PREPARATION TIME: 20 minutes
INGREDIENTS:
Ground flaxseed 1 tablespoon
Water 3 tablespoons or
Egg 1 large
Roasted almond butter ½ cup
Coconut sugar ½ cup

PALEO COOKIES, OVER 30 HEALTHY & DELICIOUS GLUTEN FREE COOKIES DESSERT RECIPES

Vanilla extract ½ teaspoon
Baking soda ¼ teaspoon
Salt 1/8 teaspoon
Chopped cranberries (frozen) ¼ cup
Chocolate chips ¼ cup

METHOD:

1. Preheat the oven to a temperature of 350 degrees Fahrenheit.
2. Take a cookie sheet and line it with parchment paper. Alternatively, you can also grease it using cooking spray.
3. Put flaxseed in a small bowl and whisk them using water to form "flax egg". It will form into a gel after five minutes. You can also use egg in place of water.
4. Take another bowl and mix coconut sugar, almond butter, baking soda, vanilla extract and salt. Combine the ingredients well.
5. Put chocolate chips and chopped cranberries in the mixture. Add the flax egg as well. Combine well.
6. When the dough is properly formed, make balls of equal size and place them on the baking sheet. You can moist your hands with water if you feel that the dough is too sticky or moist.
7. Place the baking sheet into the oven and cook for 13 minutes. Let them cool on the baking dish before placing them on a cooling rack.
8. When the cookies reach room temperature, serve.

Chocolate Chip Double Almond Cookies

Flax egg has tremendous health benefits. You can add it to any cookie recipe you like to obtain its goodness.

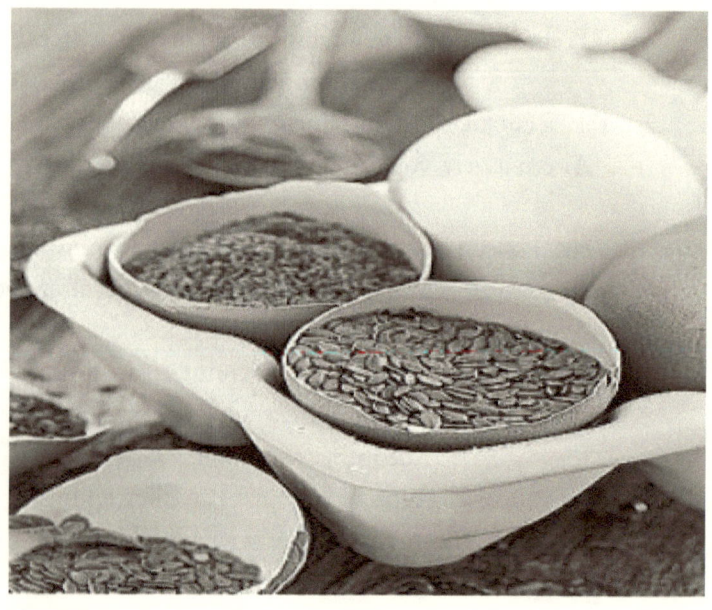

SERVES: 15
PREPARATION TIME: 1 hour
INGREDIENTS:
Ground flaxseeds 1 tablespoon
Water 3 tablespoons
Coconut sugar 1 cup
Almond butter (unsalted, roasted) 1 cup
Vanilla extract 1 teaspoon

Espresso powder 1 teaspoon
Salt ½ teaspoon
Coconut flour ¼ cup
Baking powder 1 teaspoon
Dark chocolate chips ½ cup

METHOD:

1. Preheat the oven to a temperature of 350 degrees Fahrenheit.
2. Put flaxseeds in a small bowl and whisk them using water to form "flax egg". It will form into a gel after five minutes. You can also use egg in place of water.
3. Take a large bowl and put coconut sugar, flax egg, almond butter, espresso powder, vanilla extract, and salt. Combine well.
4. Add baking powder and coconut flour gradually to form a soft dough.
5. Add chocolate chips.
6. Make balls of the size of a heaping tablespoon.
7. Place the balls on a baking sheet. Flatten them using your palm.
8. Use plastic wrap to cover the baking tray. Keep it in the refrigerator for 60 minutes.
9. Take out the baking dish and remove the plastic sheet.
10. Put the dish into the oven and cook for 7-8 minutes. The cookies should become golden brown.
11. Let them cool on the baking tray before you transfer them to the cooling rack.

Chocolate and Bacon Cookies

Feel free to experiment with this lovely recipe. Substitute some ingredients here and there and you will still end up with delicious cookies.

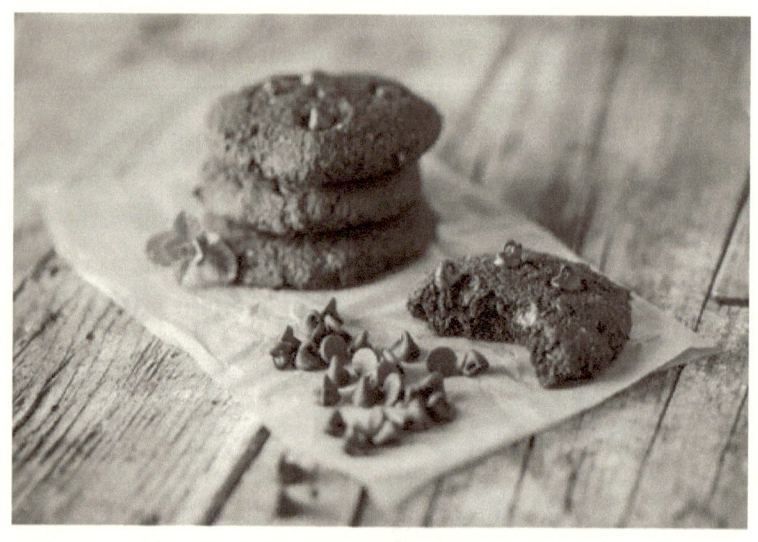

SERVES: 2-3
PREPARATION TIME: 20-25 minutes
INGREDIENTS:
Almond flour 1 cup
Salt 1/8 teaspoon
Baking soda 1/8 teaspoon
Coconut oil (melted) 3 tablespoons
Honey 2 tablespoons
Vanilla extract 1 teaspoon
Coconut or almond milk 1 teaspoon

PALEO COOKIES, OVER 30 HEALTHY & DELICIOUS GLUTEN FREE COOKIES DESSERT RECIPES

Dark chocolate (chopped) ¼ cup
Bacon (cooked, crumbled) 2-3 tablespoons/ 2 slices

METHOD:

1. Preheat the oven to a temperature of 350 degrees Fahrenheit.
2. Take a cookie sheet and line it with parchment paper.
3. Take a bowl and combine salt, baking soda and almond flour. Mix well.
4. Put all the wet ingredients in a separate bowl and whisk them together.
5. Add bacon and chocolate to the bowl of dry ingredients. Pour wet ingredients over them. Combine them well using a spatula.
6. Wet your hands and make balls of about 1.5 heaped tablespoons.
7. Place the balls on the baking sheet and press them using your palm.
8. Put the baking sheet into the preheated oven and cook for 10-12 minutes.
9. Let them cool for 3-5 minutes.
10. While the cookies are still soft, sprinkle with a little sea salt.
11. Place the cookies on the wire rack.

Cookie Dough Paleo Bites

What else do you need from a cookie recipe when it does not need baking? You save all the effort of baking and still get to enjoy the treat.

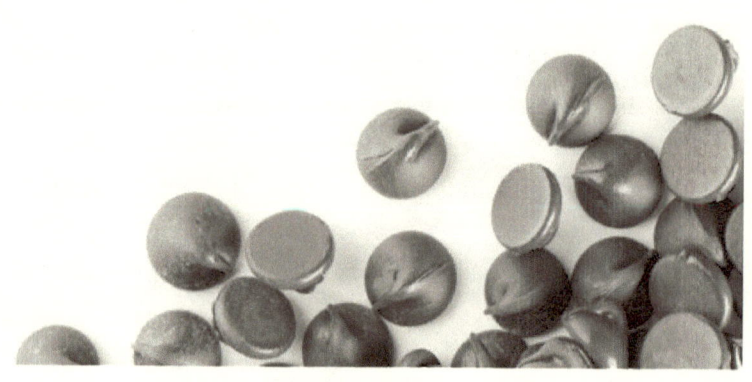

SERVES: 2-3
PREPARATION TIME: 20 minutes
INGREDIENTS:
Melted coconut oil 3 tablespoons
Full fat coconut milk 1.5 tablespoons
Vanilla extract ¾ tablespoons
Raw honey 2 tablespoons
Almond flour (blanched) ¾ cup
Chocolate chips 3 tablespoons
Chocolate chips 1 tablespoon (for drizzling)

PALEO COOKIES, OVER 30 HEALTHY & DELICIOUS GLUTEN FREE COOKIES DESSERT RECIPES

METHOD:

1. Take a cookie sheet and line it with parchment paper.
2. Take a medium sized bowl and put coconut milk, coconut oil, honey and vanilla.
3. Use a rubber spatula to mix the almond flour into the ingredients in the bowl. Combine them well. Do not over mix the batter or it may become oily.
4. Add chocolate chips and fold them in the batter.
5. Keep the dough in the refrigerator for 30 minutes.
6. Roll the dough into tablespoon-sized balls. Place them on the baking sheet.
7. Melt some chocolate chips using double boiler method over simmering water.
8. Drizzle melted chocolate over the cookies.
9. Refrigerate for a while and then serve.

Paleo Oreos

Now you do not have to stop your kids from eating the whole packet of Oreos. You can hand over a bunch of these homemade Paleo Oreos to them! They will be eating something healthier and enjoying it as well.

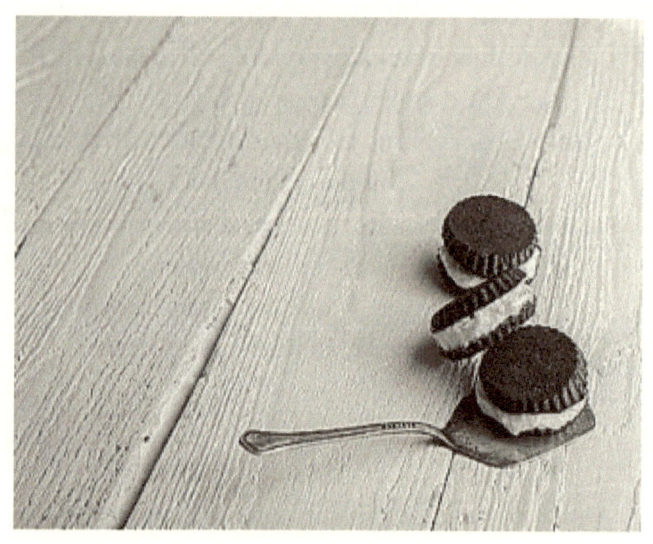

SERVES: 2-3
PREPARATION TIME: 20 minutes
INGREDIENTS (for cookies):
Almond flour (blanched) ½ cup
Arrowroot powder ¼ cup
Cacao powder (raw) ¼ cup
Butter (at room temperature) 4 tablespoons
Full fat canned coconut milk 1 tablespoon
Vanilla extract ½ teaspoon

Raw honey 2 tablespoon

INGREDIENTS (for buttercream filling):

Melted coconut butter 3 tablespoons

Vanilla extract ½ teaspoon

Water 2 tablespoons

Raw honey 1 tablespoon

METHOD (for cookies):

1. Mix arrowroot powder, cacao powder and almond flour in a medium bowl.
2. Add wet ingredients to this mixture. Combine them well and put it in the refrigerator for 15 minutes.
3. Take another bowl and mix coconut milk, butter, raw honey and vanilla extract.
4. Take the bowl out of the refrigerator and make a ball of the dough. Roll the ball between 2 parchment paper sheets. The thickness of the dough should be around 1/8 inch.
5. Remove the top sheet of the parchment paper. Transfer the lower sheet along with dough onto a baking sheet.
6. Cut out 2-inch cookies using a cookie cutter and remove the remaining dough. It can be used for making more cookies.
7. Bake the cookies in the oven at 350 degrees Fahrenheit for 10-11 minutes. They should become light golden in color.
8. Take the baking sheet out and let the cookies cool. After a few minutes, place them on a cooling rack.

METHOD (for buttercream filling):

1. Mix the ingredients of the buttercream and combine them well in the small jar of your mixer.
2. Put about 1 teaspoon of buttercream in the center of one cookie. Place another cookie on top and press them together gently.
3. Serve when they cool down.
4. Store the remaining cookies at room temperature.

Chocolate Chunk Sunbutter Cookies

Butter made from sunflower seeds is perfect for satiating your taste buds as well as for reaping health benefits. It's used in this recipe to make some amazing cookies.

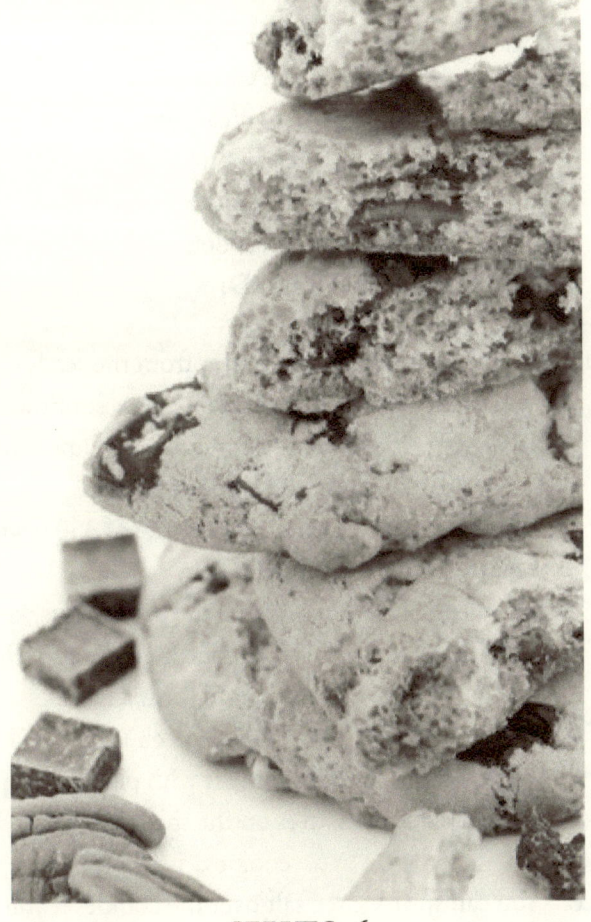

SERVES: 6
PREPARATION TIME: ½ hour

EMILY SIMMONS

INGREDIENTS:

Sunflower seed butter ½ cup
Almond butter ½ cup
Beaten egg 1
Vanilla extract 2 teaspoon
Maple syrup 1/3 cup
Cinnamon ½ teaspoon
Baking soda ½ teaspoon
Baking powder ½ teaspoon
Salt ¼ teaspoon
Chopped dark chocolate 1 cup
Sea salt 1 teaspoon

METHOD:

1. You can make sunflower butter from the seeds yourself if you do not want to buy it. Put 2 cups sunflower seeds in a jar of your food processor. Process it until you get a creamy and smooth butter.
2. Preheat the oven to a temperature of 350 degrees Fahrenheit.
3. Take a large bowl and mix all the ingredients, keeping aside chocolate chunks. Mix the ingredients well until they are combined to form a batter.
4. Fold in the chocolate chunks.
5. Take a baking sheet and line it with parchment paper. Scoop out the batter on the sheet and make six cookies.
6. You can sprinkle sea salt over the cookies if you like.
7. Put the baking sheet into the oven and cook for about 18-20 minutes. They should become golden brown.

8. Let them cool and then serve.

<u>Pumpkin Cake Chocolate Cookies</u>

You might have become bored with all these similar-looking cookie recipes. Here, we have a break in the monotony for you. These pumpkin cookies are a combination of cake and cookies. They are softer on the top and crisp at the bottom. Enjoy!

EMILY SIMMONS

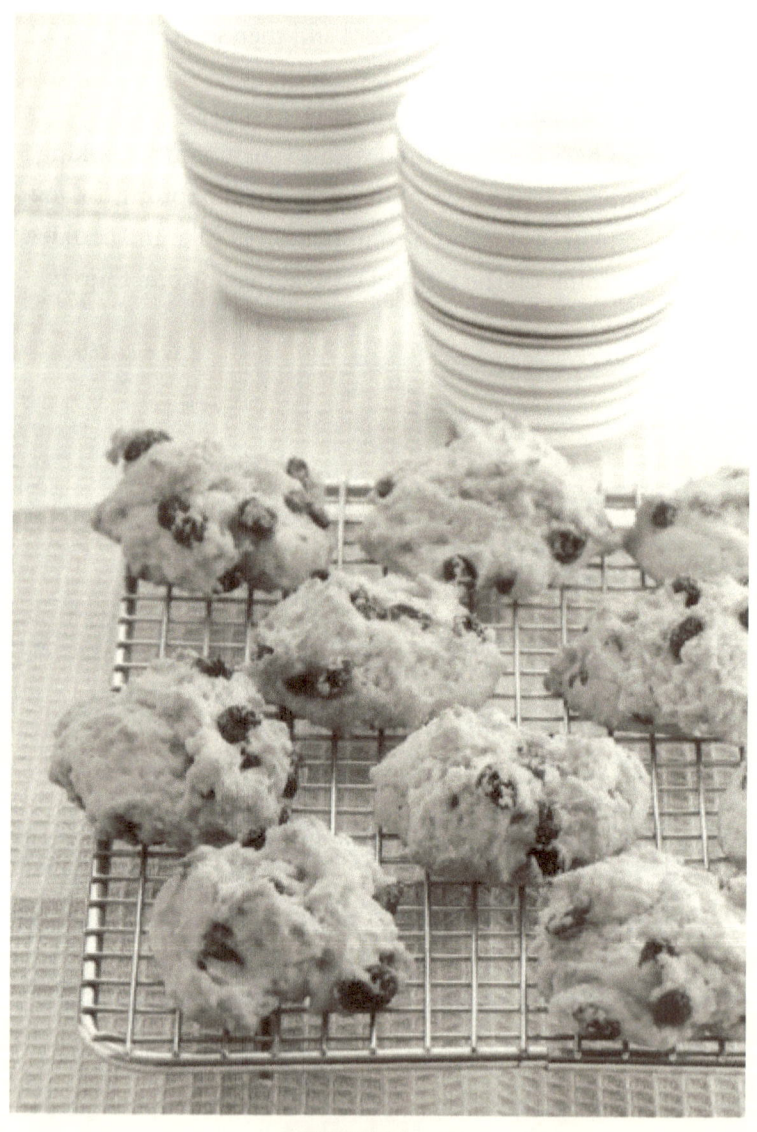

SERVES: 20
PREPARATION TIME: 20 minutes
INGREDIENTS:

PALEO COOKIES, OVER 30 HEALTHY & DELICIOUS GLUTEN FREE COOKIES DESSERT RECIPES

Pumpkin/sweet potato/banana puree ¾ cups
Coconut flour ½ cup
Melted coconut oil ½ cup
Eggs 6
Vanilla extract 2 teaspoons
Honey ¼ cup
Cinnamon 1 teaspoon
Nutmeg 1 teaspoon
Allspice mix 1 teaspoon
Baking powder ½ teaspoon
Chocolate chips 1 cup

METHOD:

1. Preheat the oven to a temperature of 350 degrees Fahrenheit.
2. Take the jar of your electric mixer and put in coconut oil, pumpkin, honey, eggs and vanilla. Process to combine the ingredients.
3. In a bowl, sieve cinnamon powder, nutmeg, coconut flour, baking powder and allspice mix.
4. Add this flour to the mixer jar and process to combine them. There should be no clumps in the batter.
5. Add chocolate chips and fold them in the batter,
6. Take a baking sheet and line it with parchment paper.
7. Scoop out the dough around the size of a large tablespoon on the baking sheet.
8. Put the sheet in the oven to cook for 11-12 minutes. The bottoms should be cooked in this time.
9. You will find these cookies are not like normal ones. The upper crust should be softer and the bottom

harder.

10. Take them out of the oven and let cool slightly.

11. Serve warm.

12. You can store them in an airtight jar for 3 days.

Grain Free Chocolate Bars

The goodness of walnuts along with the taste of chocolate is a perfect combination. Just a little innovation in the shape of cakes, cookies and bars can add a new touch of fun to your breakfast.

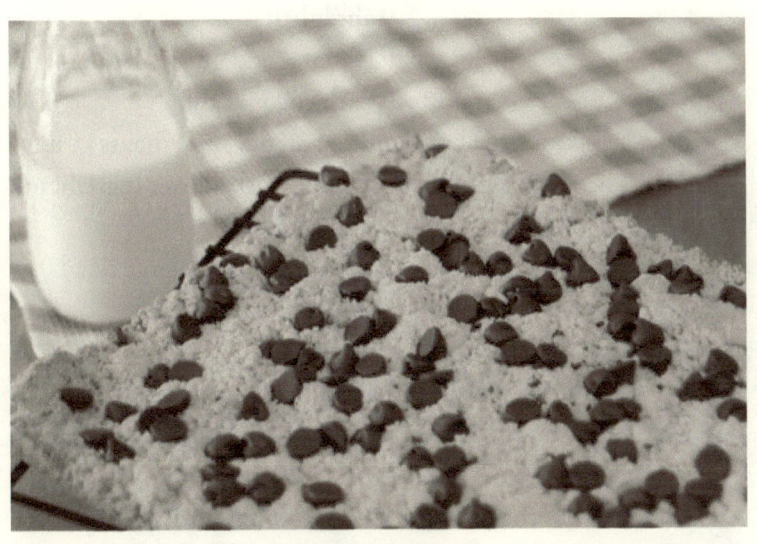

SERVES: 4-5
PREPARATION TIME: 40-50 minutes
INGREDIENTS:
Almond flour (blanched) 2.5 cups
Baking soda 1 teaspoon
Sea salt ½ teaspoon
Honey 1/3 cup
Brown eggs 2 large
Melted coconut oil ¼ cup

Vanilla extract 2 teaspoons
Almond milk 1 tablespoon
Chocolate chips (semi-sweet) ¾ cup
Walnuts ¼ cup

METHOD:

1. Preheat the oven to a temperature of 350 degrees Fahrenheit.
2. Take an 8" baking pan (square) and grease its sides and bottom with coconut oil.
3. Take a large bowl and put all dry ingredients in it.
4. Take another small bowl and whisk all wet ingredients together with a hand whisk.
5. Now pour the wet mixture into the large bowl containing dry ingredients. Combine them using the hand blender.
6. Add chocolate chips and fold them in the batter.
7. Pour the batter into the greased baking pan. Spread it evenly using a spatula.
8. Put it in the oven for 20-25 minutes until the top crust is cooked and golden brown.
9. Take out of the oven and let cool for 10-15 minutes.
10. Cut the cake carefully into bars.
11. Store the bars in an airtight container in the refrigerator.
12. Microwave to warm up before serving.

Vegan Chocolate Cookies

These light and crumbly cookies have yummy chocolate chunks inside them. If you enjoy larger bits of chocolate in your sweets, this recipe is for you.

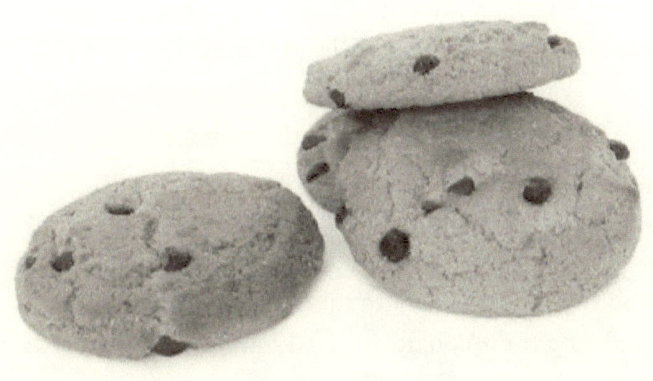

SERVES: 4-5
PREPARATION TIME: 30-40 minutes
INGREDIENTS:
Almond meal 1 cup
Sea salt ¼ teaspoon
Baking soda 1/8 teaspoon
Cinnamon ¼ teaspoon
Melted butter or coconut oil 3 tablespoons
Maple syrup or honey 2 tablespoons
Vanilla extract 1.5 teaspoons
Water 0.5-1 teaspoon

Dark chocolate, chopped/ chocolate chips 3-4 tablespoons

METHOD:

1. Preheat the oven to a temperature of 350 degrees Fahrenheit.
2. Take a medium sized bowl and put in salt, almond meal, cinnamon and baking soda. Mix them well.
3. Take another bowl and mix maple syrup/ honey, coconut oil and vanilla extract.
4. Pour these wet ingredients into the other bowl. Add enough water to bind the ingredients together.
5. Add chopped chocolate pieces and stir in.
6. Take a baking sheet and line it with parchment paper.
7. Scoop out 2 tablespoonfuls of batter for each cookie onto the baking sheet.
8. Bake the cookies for 10-12 minutes until the edges become golden.
9. Take out the baking sheet and let the cookies cool.
10. Take them out and enjoy!

PALEO COOKIES, OVER 30 HEALTHY & DELICIOUS GLUTEN FREE COOKIES DESSERT RECIPES

Gluten Free Cookies

A ball of chocolate-packed cookie, when it crumbles in your mouth, does not leave you any option but to think of heaven. Indulge in the crime of gobbling these cookies down. Shhhhhh! Do not tell your mom!

SERVES: 15

PREPARATION TIME: 25-30 minutes

INGREDIENTS:

Softened coconut butter ¾ cup

Brown sugar ¾ cup

Coconut oil 3 tablespoons

Large eggs 2

Baking soda ½ teaspoon

Kosher salt ½ teaspoon

Almond flour 3 cups

Chocolate chips 6 ounces

METHOD:

1. Preheat the oven to a temperature of 350 degrees Fahrenheit.
2. Soften the coconut butter. Combine it with coconut oil and brown sugar. Beat the ingredients for 2-3 minutes in a mixer with paddle attachment.
3. Add an egg to the mixture. When the egg is fully mixed, add the other egg. Now, add kosher salt and baking soda.
4. Pulse the mixture on a medium-low speed. Gradually add almond flour to avoid making lumps. Mix them well.
5. Add chocolate chips and fold them completely.
6. Make balls of about 2 tablespoons of the dough using your hands. Put the balls on a baking sheet. You can flatten them if you like.
7. Bake them for 10-11 minutes until the balls become light brown on the top.
8. Take the cookies out of the oven and let cool. Serve after 5-10 minutes.

Cut Out Grain Free Cookies

The icing on top just provides the finishing touch to these delicious cookies.

SERVES: 10-12

PREPARATION TIME: 1 hour

INGREDIENTS (for cookies):

Almond flour, blanched 2 cups

Sea salt ¼ teaspoon

Baking soda ¼ teaspoon

Coconut oil, virgin, melted ¼ cup

Honey ¼ cup

Vanilla extract 1 tablespoon

INGREDIENTS (for icing):

Chilled coconut milk, full fat 1 can

Honey 1 tablespoon

METHOD (for cookies):

1. Preheat the oven to a temperature of 350 degrees Fahrenheit.
2. Take a medium sized bowl and mix baking soda, salt and almond flour.
3. Take a small bowl and whisk honey, coconut oil, vanilla extract, and honey together.
4. Add the whisked mixture to the bowl of flour and blend together until you get a smooth paste.
5. Take a large baking sheet and line it with parchment paper.
6. Roll the dough between two parchment paper sheets.

The thickness should be about ¼ inches. Freeze the dough for 5 minutes after rolling out. This makes it easy to cut.

7. Cut out the cookies using cookie cutters and place them on the baking sheet.
8. Freeze the cut out cookies for 5 minutes so that they can hold their shape during baking.
9. Bake them for 10-12 minutes. The cookies will become golden brown at the edges.
10. Take them out and let cool for a few minutes, then place on cooling racks.
11. Repeat the procedure for the remaining dough.

METHOD (for icing):

1. Scoop out coconut cream from the can into a small bowl. Keep the remaining milk for making smoothies later.
2. Pour honey over coconut cream and whisk until smooth. Transfer the mixture into a piping bag. Pipe the cream on the cookies after they have cooled down. Keep the remaining cream in an airtight jar and store in a refrigerator.

Paleo Macadamia Cookies

You might have become bored of eating dark chocolate. Here we have macadamia nut cookies for you to give to your taste buds a change.

SERVES: 4-5
PREPARATION TIME: 45 minutes
INGREDIENTS:

Macadamia nuts, raw, whole ¾ cups
Almond flour 1 cup
Desiccated coconut, unsweetened 1 cup
Ground ginger 1 teaspoon
Honey ¼ cup
Melted Coconut oil ¼ cup
Baking soda ½ teaspoon
Water, divided 2 tablespoons

METHOD:

1. Preheat the oven to a temperature of 320 degrees Fahrenheit.
2. Spread macadamia nuts on the baking sheet. Bake for 5-7 minutes and roast them slightly. Chop the nuts roughly when they're slightly cool.
3. Reduce the heat of the oven to 250 degrees Fahrenheit.
4. Take a large bowl and mix desiccated coconut, almond flour, ginger and macadamia nuts.
5. Take a saucepan and pour in coconut oil and honey. Melt them gently.
6. Take a small bowl and mix water (1 tablespoon), and

baking soda. Add this mixture to the coconut oil mixture.

7. When you see the mixture frothing up, take the saucepan off from the heat. Pour the ingredients onto the wet ingredients. Add 1 more tablespoon of water into this mixture and combine well.

8. Take a baking sheet and line it with parchment paper.

9. Take an ice cream scoop and make 12 cookies or more if you have more batter.

10. Place the cookies on the baking sheet. Flatten the cookies using the back side of the scoop.

11. Put the sheet into the oven and bake for 22-25 minutes. The cookies will become golden brown.

12. Take out the cookies and let them cool. Serve.

Brownie Bites

Baking is eliminated, but taste is not! These cookie balls are just so easy to make and taste equally as good. These little cookie balls are bound to be a hit with the whole family. Serve them as after dinner truffles if you like, too.

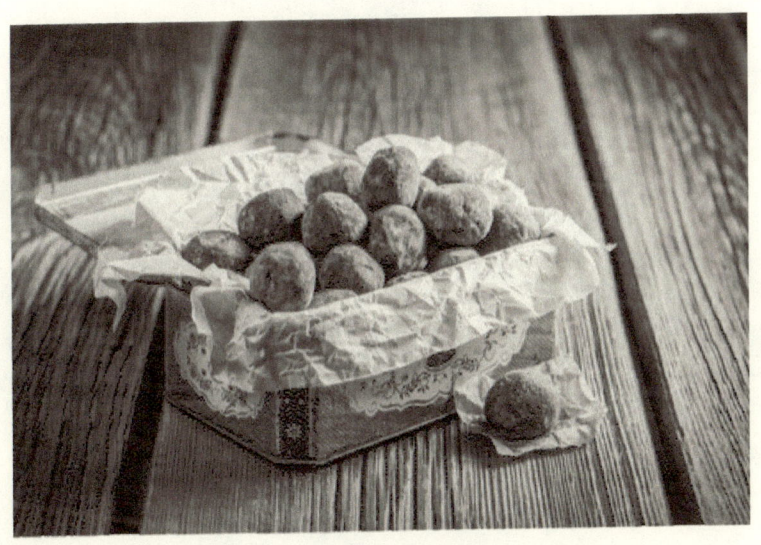

SERVES: 4-5
PREPARATION TIME: 45 minutes
INGREDIENTS:
Walnut halves 1.5 cups
Cocoa powder ¼ cup
Vanilla extract 1 teaspoon
Sea salt ¼ teaspoon
Pitted soft dates 10
Water 1 tablespoon

Cocoa powder to coat

METHOD:

1. Take the jar of food processor with "S" blade. Grind the walnut halves into a smooth meal.
2. Put the remaining ingredients in the jar. Process until a sticky dough is formed. The dough should be uniform in consistency.
3. Take a baking sheet and line it with parchment paper.
4. Scoop out heaped teaspoons of dough.
5. Roll the dough into balls, using your hands. Roll the cookies in cocoa powder.
6. Refrigerate the cookie balls and serve chilled.

Banana Bread Chocolate Cookies

SERVES: 4-5
PREPARATION TIME: 20-25 minutes
INGREDIENTS:
Eggs 2
Softened Butter 1.5 tablespoons
Mashed banana ½ cup
Almond milk ¼ cup
Honey ¼ cup
Vanilla 1 teaspoon
Coconut flour ½ cup
Cinnamon ½ tablespoon
Baking powder 1 teaspoon
Sea salt 1/8 teaspoon
Dark chocolate chips ½ cup

METHOD:

1. Preheat the oven to a temperature of 350 degrees Fahrenheit.
2. Mix butter, eggs, banana, honey, vanilla and almond milk in a bowl.
3. Take another bowl and mix cinnamon, coconut flour, salt and baking powder. Add this mixture to the other bowl. Combine all the ingredients well.
4. Put in chocolate chips and fold them in well.
5. Take a baking sheet and line it with parchment paper.
6. Take out a spoonful of batter for each cookie, place on the baking sheet, and flatten them with the back side of the spoon.
7. Put the baking sheet into the oven and cook for 18-20 minutes.
8. Remove from oven and let cool for 5 minutes. Transfer the banana cookies onto a cooling rack.
9. Serve.

Sugar Lemon Cookies

You can experiment with the look and feel of these wonderful lemon cookies. Eat them as single cookies or join two together with lemon curd- just as you like. They will taste awesome either way.

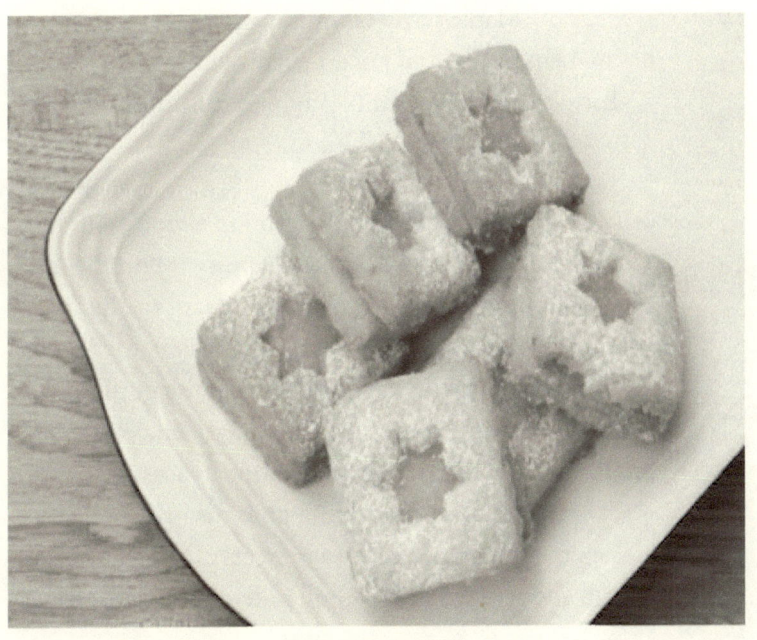

SERVES: 3-4
PREPARATION TIME: 25 minutes
INGREDIENTS (for cookies):
Ground almonds 2 cups
Arrowroot powder 1 tablespoon
Baking soda ¼ teaspoon
Salt ¼ teaspoon

Melted coconut oil ¼ cup
Maple syrup ¼ cup
Vanilla extract 1 tablespoon
Lemon zest 1 small lemon
INGREDIENTS (for lemon curd):
Water 60 milliliters
Arrowroot powder 3 tablespoons
Maple syrup 60 milliliters
Lemon zest and juice 1 small lemon
Turmeric or yellow edible color ½ teaspoon
METHOD (for cookies):

1. Put arrowroot powder and ground almonds in the food processor. Process to make powdery flour. Sieve the flour into a medium bowl. Discard the lumps.
2. Pour maple syrup, coconut oil, lemon zest and vanilla extract into the food processor. Pulse until the ingredients are combined well.
3. Return the sifted flour to the food processor. Pulse until a smooth dough is formed.
4. Pack the dough between two sheets of cling film. Roll it till about ½ cm thick. Chill in the refrigerator for 20 minutes.
5. Preheat the oven to a temperature of 338 degrees Fahrenheit and line a baking sheet with parchment paper.
6. Remove the dough from the refrigerator and roll it between two sheets of parchment paper.
7. Cut out cookies using cookie cutters. Cut half of the cookies full in shape and half of them with the center

cut out.

8. Place them on the baking tray and cook for 8-10 minutes. Do not let the cookies brown excessively.

9. Let them cool on a wire rack before joining together with lemon curd.

1.

METHOD (for lemon curd):

1. Mix arrowroot powder and water in a saucepan. Dissolve the powder properly in the water.
2. Heat it over medium heat and bring the mixture to boil. The mixture will thicken gradually while you stir.
3. Drizzle maple syrup in gradually and cook on medium heat for a minute.
4. Take the saucepan off the heat and pour the mixture in a plastic bowl. Put in lemon zest and juice and mix. Add turmeric or yellow color and combine the ingredients.
5. Let it cool, and whisk before serving. When the spread is ready, spread on the whole cookies and top with the ones that are cut out in the center. You can refrigerate the lemon curd in the refrigerator for 3 days.

PALEO COOKIES, OVER 30 HEALTHY & DELICIOUS GLUTEN FREE COOKIES DESSERT RECIPES

1.

Thumbprint Blueberry Cookies

The jelly-like texture of the filling in these thumbprint blueberry cookies is just so good that you'll want to have more than two at a time! Blueberries are good for you, so that's alright.

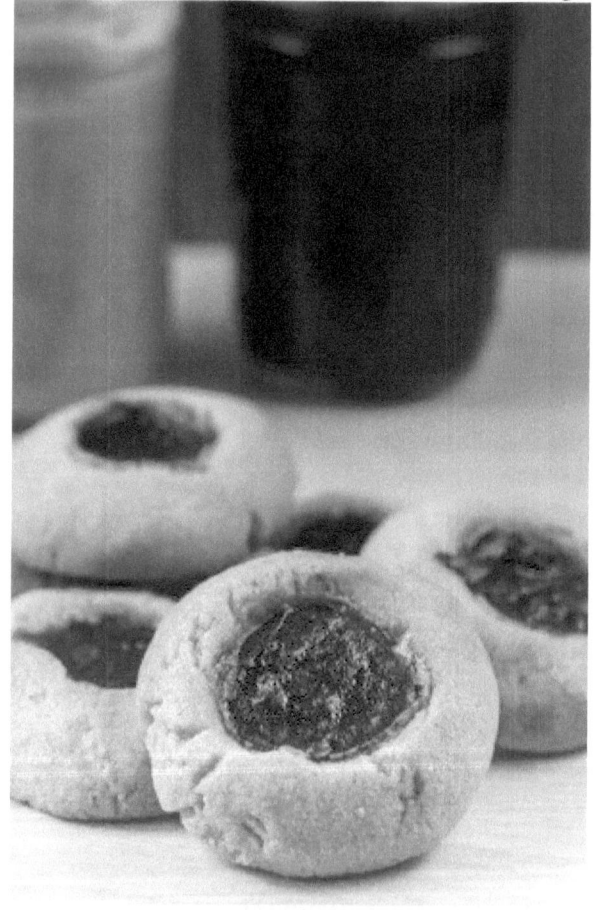

SERVES: 10
PREPARATION TIME: 35 minutes
INGREDIENTS (for filling):
Blueberries 2 cups

Maple syrup 1 tablespoon

Water ¼ cup

Lemon juice ¼ cup

Nutmeg ½ teaspoon

Cinnamon 1 teaspoon

Arrowroot powder 1-2 tablespoon

INGREDIENTS (for cookies):

Almond flour, blanched 2 cups

Arrowroot powder 1 cup

Arrowroot powder 1/2 cup (dusting)

Salt 1 teaspoon

Vanilla extract 1 teaspoon

Maple syrup 1/3 cup

Melted coconut oil, organic ¼ cup

METHOD (for filling):

1. To prepare filling, heat a saucepan over medium heat and put in maple syrup, blueberries, lemon juice, water, cinnamon and nutmeg.
2. Stir continuously and let the mixture boil. You can a use a wooden spatula to mash the berries.
3. When you see the liquid reducing, turn down the heat and put in the arrowroot powder. Let the filling thicken, stirring continuously.
4. Remove the saucepan from the heat and let the mixture cool. You can add more blueberries to the filling mixture at this stage if you want.

1.

METHOD (for cookies):

1. Preheat the oven to a temperature of 350 degrees Fahrenheit.
2. Take a large bowl and mix arrowroot powder, salt and almond flour.
3. Add vanilla extract, coconut oil and maple syrup. Combine all the ingredients well and make a dough ball. You can make the dough using your hands as well.
4. Take a baking sheet and line it with parchment paper.
5. Make small balls of the dough and place on the baking sheet. Use all the dough. You can use arrowroot powder for dusting if you find the dough is too sticky.
6. Press your thumb in the middle of the rolled cookies to make a well.
7. Put about a tablespoon of blueberry filling into the well in the center.
8. Place the baking sheet in the oven and bake for 20 minutes.
9. Take out the cookies and let cool.
10. You can keep the remaining filling for using it in other recipes.

Pecan Pumpkin Cookies

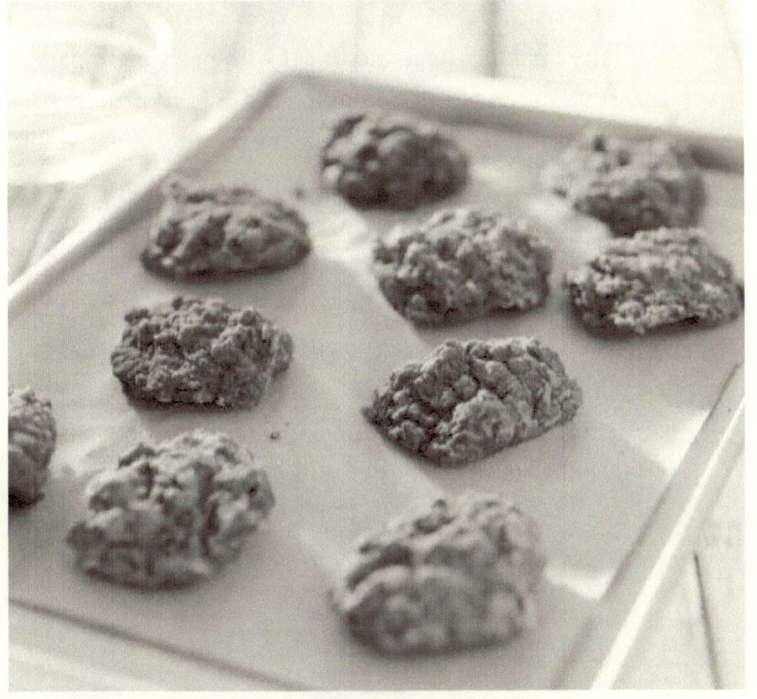

SERVES: 2-3
PREPARATION TIME: 10 minutes
INGREDIENTS:

Pecans 1/3 cup

Almonds ¼ cup

Pitted dates ¾ cup (8 large)

Ground flaxseed ¼ cup

Canned pumpkin 3 tablespoons

Vanilla 1 teaspoon

Pumpkin pie spice 1.5 teaspoon

Cinnamon ½ teaspoon

Salt a pinch

METHOD:

1. Take a baking sheet and line it with parchment paper.
2. Put almonds and pecans in a jar of food processor. Pulse until the mixture forms fine crumbs. Remove and place in a medium bowl.
3. Put dates in the food processor and pulse to make a smooth paste.
4. Return the mixture of processed nuts to the food processor with the dates. Add the remaining ingredients and pulse to combine everything well.
5. Remove the dough and make a large ball. Now, make 8 balls out of the dough and flatten them to make cookies.
6. Refrigerate for a while and serve cold.

Cashew Cardamom Date Balls

When your kids come rushing home from school and ask for something to eat immediately, just ask them to wait for 10 minutes and quickly make them these quick cashew balls. Apart from the health benefits of dates and cashews, these balls taste amazing too.

SERVES: 2-3

PREPARATION TIME: 10 minutes

INGREDIENTS:

Cashews 1 cup

Pitted medjool dates 1 cup

Orange zest 1 orange

Cardamom ¼ teaspoon

Coconut flakes 1/3 cup

METHOD:

1. Leaving coconut aside, put all the ingredients in the food processor. Pulse until all the components are combined well.
2. Make balls of the mixture about the size of a tablespoon.
3. Roll the balls in coconut flakes. If you find that the coconut flakes are not sticking to the balls, you can use a little water to coat them.
4. Serve fresh.

EMILY SIMMONS

<u>Carrot Cake Cookies</u>

The goodness of carrots with the amazing taste of chocolate is just what you need during winter. Have these cookies with a glass of organic milk or a smoothie, and your healthy tasty breakfast is done!

SERVES: 4-5

PREPARATION TIME: 50 minutes

INGREDIENTS:

Shredded carrots 2 large

Coconut sugar 1 cup

Coconut oil, melted 1 cup

Whisked eggs 2

Vanilla extract 1 teaspoon

Coconut flour 1 cup

Tapioca flour ½ cup

Pumpkin pie spice ½ teaspoon

Chocolate chunks 1 cup

METHOD:

1. Preheat the oven to a temperature of 350 degrees Fahrenheit.
2. Take a bowl large enough to accommodate carrots, coconut oil, coconut sugar, vanilla extract and eggs. Whisk the ingredients and combine them well.
3. Add tapioca flour, coconut flour, salt and pumpkin spice. Mix them and combine.
4. Add chocolate chunks in the mixture and fold them in. You might find the dough a little dry and hard. The cookies will be fine after baking.
5. Take a baking sheet and line it with parchment paper.

6. Take an ice cream scoop and take out 12-13 scoops of the dough onto the baking dish. Press down the cookies using your fingers.
7. Put the baking tray in the oven and cook for 35-40 minutes. The cookies should be cooked through.

Ginger Cookies

Ginger gives cookies a deliciously warm, tangy flavor. If you are a fan of ginger, this recipe will be a winner for you.

SERVES: 12

PREPARATION TIME: 50 minutes

INGREDIENTS:

Almond flour 1.5 cups

Softened coconut oil 2 tablespoons

Maple syrup ¼ cup

Blackstrap molasses 1 tablespoon

Ground ginger 2 teaspoons

Sea salt 1/8 teaspoon

Baking soda ¼ teaspoon

METHOD:

1. Put all the ingredients in a bowl. Mix to combine them well.
2. Refrigerate the mixture for 30 minutes. It should become firm before you take it out of the fridge.
3. Preheat the oven to a temperature of 350 degrees Fahrenheit.
4. Take a baking sheet and line it with parchment paper.
5. Scoop out balls of dough onto the baking dish. You can flatten the balls using a fork till you reach the desired thickness.
6. Put the baking sheet in the oven and cook for 8-10 minutes. They will become firm around the edges, but will remain soft in the center.
7. Take out the sheet and let them cool for 10 minutes.
8. Transfer the cookies on a cooling rack and then serve.

PALEO COOKIES, OVER 30 HEALTHY & DELICIOUS GLUTEN FREE COOKIES DESSERT RECIPES

Pumpkin Pie Cookies

These cookies might become your favorite once you have them. Have them for breakfast or after lunch, the soft cookies will please you anytime.

SERVES: 24

PREPARATION TIME: 25 minutes

INGREDIENTS:

Almond butter, creamy 1 cup

Pumpkin puree ½ cup

Maple syrup ¼ cup

Pumpkin pie spice 2 teaspoons

Sea salt ¼ teaspoon

Dark chocolate chips ½ cup

METHOD:

1. Preheat the oven to a temperature of 350 degrees Fahrenheit.
2. Take a baking sheet and line it with parchment paper.
3. In a medium sized bowl, put all the ingredients and mix them to form a thick batter.
4. Put in the chocolate chips and fold them into the batter.
5. Since you are not putting eggs in this recipe, you can taste it to test at any point of time and adjust the ingredients accordingly.
6. Drop a tablespoon or a scoop of the batter for each cookie onto the baking sheet. Use a wet fork to press the cookies down a little.
7. Bake them for 12-15 minutes until you see the edges becoming golden.

8. Take the sheet out of the oven and let cool.
9. Chill the cookies before serving.

Banana Bacon Cookies

Bananas make these cookies melt in your mouth. The softness is unparalleled to any other cookies. Moreover, there is bacon to enhance the taste.

SERVES: 3-4

PREPARATION TIME: 30 minutes

INGREDIENTS:

Mashed bananas 2 small

Sunflower seed butter 1 cup

Honey ½ cup

Whisked egg 1

Vanilla extract 1 teaspoon

Cinnamon ¼ teaspoon

Baking soda ½ teaspoon

Baking powder ½ teaspoon

Salt a pinch

Chocolate chips ½ cup

Cooked and diced bacon 3 strips

EMILY SIMMONS

METHOD:

1. Preheat the oven to a temperature of 350 degrees Fahrenheit.
2. Take a baking sheet and line it with parchment paper.
3. Take a medium sized bowl and put in butter, banana, egg, honey, and vanilla. Mix them well.
4. Add baking powder, baking soda, salt and cinnamon. Mix well.
5. Put bacon and chocolate chips into the mixture and fold them through properly.
6. Scoop out tablespoons of batter onto the baking sheet. Leave some room between each cookie to allow them to spread out. The batter will make about 12 cookies.
7. Put the tray in the oven and cook for 20 minutes. Take it out and let cool.
8. Serve.

Macadamia Nut Cookies

Macadamia nuts always taste good, and they're especially yummy when combined with chocolate, as in this recipe.

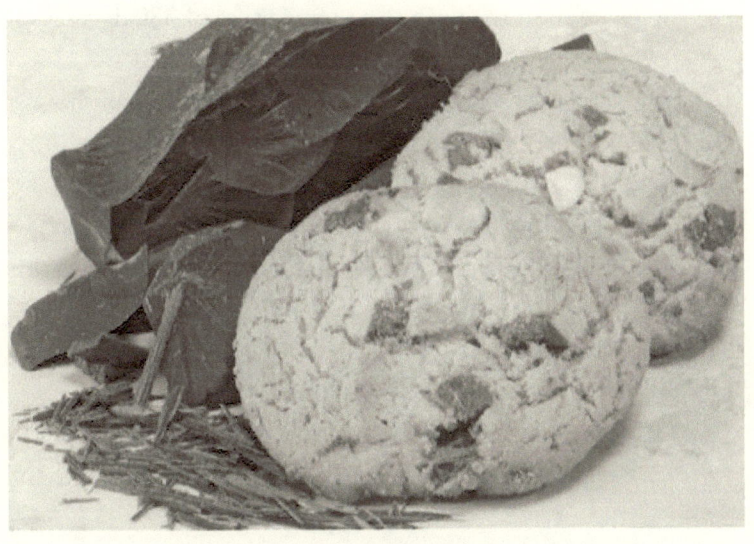

SERVES: 3-4
PREPARATION TIME: 40 minutes
INGREDIENTS:
Almond flour 2.5 cups
Coconut flour 2 tablespoons
Shredded coconut, unsweetened 2/3 cups
Baking soda 1 teaspoon
Melted coconut oil ½ cup
Melted raw honey ¼ cup
Whisked eggs 3
Vanilla extract 1 tablespoon

EMILY SIMMONS

Macadamia nuts 2/3 cup
Chocolate chips 2/3 cup
Sea salt ¼ teaspoon
METHOD:

1. Preheat the oven to a temperature of 350 degrees Fahrenheit.
2. Take a baking sheet and line it with aluminum sheets.
3. In a medium sized bowl, mix coconut flour, almond flour, sea salt, baking soda and shredded coconut.
4. Take another bowl to mix together vanilla extract, eggs, honey and coconut oil. Pour the mixture into the other bowl.
5. Add chocolate chips and macadamia nuts and fold them in the mixture.
6. Make balls about the size of 2 tablespoons of batter. Position these balls on the baking sheet and press them down using your hand.
7. Place the cookies in the oven and cook for 18-20 minutes. Check after 16 minutes that the bottom of the cookies are not overcooking or burning.
8. Let them cool after you take them out.
9. Serve and enjoy!

Orange Blossom Cookies

The tangy taste of oranges in the cookies is just so awesome. The freshness of the orange juice remains intact even after baking.

SERVES: 3-4

PREPARATION TIME: 30 minutes

INGREDIENTS:

Almond flour 3 cups

Coconut flour ¼ cup

Melted coconut oil 1/3 cup

Navel orange zest 1 large

Vanilla extract 1 tablespoon

Baking soda, aluminum free ½ teaspoon

Sea salt a pinch

Honey, local, raw 1/3 cup

Orange juice 1/3 cup (from half navel orange)

METHOD:

1. Preheat the oven to a temperature of 350 degrees Fahrenheit.
2. Take a baking sheet and line it with parchment paper.
3. Put all the ingredients in a glass bowl and mix them using a pastry blender.
4. Make a large dough ball of the mixture and place it on a piece of wax paper. Refrigerate the dough for 15 minutes.
5. Make 1.5 inch sized balls out of the dough and position them on the sheet.
6. Press down the balls using a wet fork. You can also make a pattern of cross hatching with the fork.
7. Put the baking sheet in the oven and bake the cookies for 15 minutes. The top crust of the cookies should become golden brown.
8. Take the sheet out of the oven and let cool.
9. Serve and enjoy.

Sunflower Cookies

The visual appeal as well as taste of these cookies puts them in a
class of their own. The sunflower seeds and butter give these
Paleo cookies a completely unique taste. Serve them with a cup
of coffee and enjoy the delicacy.

SERVES: 3-4

PREPARATION TIME: 30 minutes

INGREDIENTS (for cookies):

Coconut flour 6 tablespoons

Sunflower seed butter/ nut butter ½ cup

Coconut sugar 2/3 cup

Melted coconut oil 1/3 cup

Egg 1

INGREDIENTS (for decoration):

Sunflower seeds 2 tablespoons

Dark chocolate chips (optional)

12
METHOD:

1. Preheat the oven to a temperature of 350 degrees Fahrenheit.
2. Take a baking sheet and line it with parchment paper or grease the sheet.
3. In a large bowl, put egg, sunflower seed butter, coconut sugar, coconut oil and coconut flour. Mix well to combine the ingredients.
4. Keep the dough in the freezer for 10-12 minutes. This makes the dough less sticky and the cookies also spread less after freezing.
5. Put the chocolate chips and sunflower seeds in a small bowl.
6. Take the dough out from the freezer and make 12 balls out of it. Place these balls on the baking sheet. Flatten them gently.
7. Push a chocolate chip in the center of each cookie. You can avoid chocolate chips if you do not like them with sunflower seeds. Now decorate the cookies with sunflower seeds. Push the seeds gently into the cookies
8. Bake them for 12 minutes. Take the baking sheet out of the oven and let cool.
9. Serve at room temperature.

Lazy Espresso Cookies

Sometimes, you just do not have time for a proper meal during busy hours in the office. A quick shot of espresso cookies is a great way to energize you when you need a pick-me-up at the office. Just grab one of these cookies if you didn't have time to have lunch today!

SERVES: 4-5

PREPARATION TIME: 30 minutes

INGREDIENTS:

Almond flour 2 cups

Baking soda ¼ teaspoon

Salt a pinch

Cinnamon 2 dashes

Espresso powder 1-2 tablespoons

Coconut powder or shredded coconut, unsweetened ½ cup

Coconut oil 1/3 cup

Maple syrup ¼ cup

Vanilla extract 1 teaspoon

Coconut milk 1 tablespoon

Chocolate chips ¾ cup

EMILY SIMMONS

METHOD:

1. Preheat the oven to a temperature of 350 degrees Fahrenheit.
2. Take a baking sheet and line it with parchment paper.
3. In a medium sized bowl, put all the ingredients and combine them well.
4. Add chocolate chips and fold them in the batter.
5. Make balls of this dough about the size of a heaping tablespoon.
6. Place the balls in the baking sheet and flatten them using your hands. Leave a gap of about one inch between each cookie to allow them some room to spread.
7. Put the baking tray in the oven and cook for 12-15 minutes.
8. Remove the tray from the oven and let it cool for 2 minutes.
9. Transfer the cookies on the wire rack and let cool for a while.
10. Serve warm or at room temperature.

Avocado Double Chocolate Cookies

The earthy and fresh flavor of avocado seems to go with anything. Even if you combine avocado with cookies, the texture and taste comes out really well. Enjoy these cookies and save some for later as well.

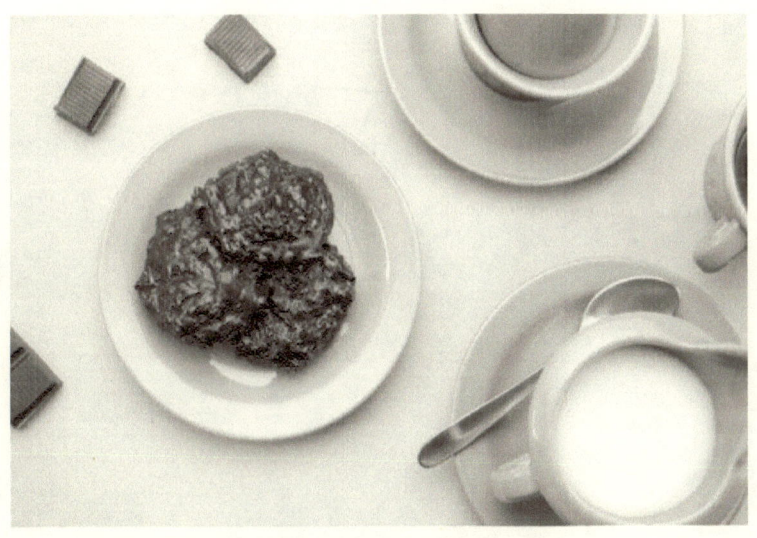

SERVES: 4-5
PREPARATION TIME: 25 minutes
INGREDIENTS:
Baking soda ½ teaspoon
Water 1 tablespoon
Avocado, very ripe 1
Maple syrup ¼ cup
Egg 1
Cocoa powder ½ cup

EMILY SIMMONS

Dark chocolate, unsweetened, chopped 1 ounce

PALEO COOKIES, OVER 30 HEALTHY & DELICIOUS GLUTEN FREE COOKIES DESSERT RECIPES

METHOD:

1. Preheat the oven to a temperature of 350 degrees Fahrenheit.
2. Take a baking sheet and line it with parchment paper and keep aside.
3. In a small bowl, mix baking soda with water and set aside.
4. Using a hand blender, whip avocado properly. Add maple syrup and continue whipping to achieve a smooth mixture.
5. Add egg and whisk again.
6. Add cocoa powder gradually and continue mixing on a medium speed of the blender.
7. Once you are done adding the ingredients mentioned, turn on the high speed and mix well. Mix baking soda mixture into this mixture and blend it well with everything else.
8. Add chopped chocolate. Stir well to combine the chocolate. The dough will be soft in texture.
9. Using an ice-cream scoop, scoop out two tablespoons sized dough on the baking sheet. Keep a gap of at least 2 inches in between the cookies. Flatten them using the back side of a spoon.
10. Bake the cookies for 8-10 minutes. It is fine if they look slightly underdone.
11. Take the baking sheet out of the oven and let it cool slightly.
12. Transfer the cookies on a wire rack and let them cool properly.

EMILY SIMMONS

13. Serve.

1.

Sandwich Cookies

This last recipe of the book is so worth the extra effort. You only need an ice cream maker at home. If you do not have it, do not worry. You can make normal cream using simple tools. Just go ahead and make these sandwich cookies. Your entire family is going to love them. Enjoy them in the evening with smoothies or coffee.

SERVES: 4-5

PREPARATION TIME: 25 minutes

INGREDIENTS (for cookies):

Almond flour 2 cups

Salt ½ teaspoon

Baking soda ½ teaspoon

Pumpkin pie spice 1 tablespoon (more for adding sprinkles)

Pumpkin puree ½ cup

Mashed and ripe banana 1 small

Maple syrup ¼ cup

Vanilla extract 1 tablespoon

Coconut oil 1/3 cup

Chocolate chips ½ cup

EMILY SIMMONS

INGREDIENTS (for cream filling):
Coconut milk 1 can
Pumpkin puree 1 can
Maple syrup ¼ cup
Pumpkin pie spice ½ tablespoon
METHOD (for cookies):

1. Preheat the oven to a temperature of 350 degrees Fahrenheit.
2. Take a baking sheet and line it with parchment paper.
3. Take a large bowl and put baking soda, almond flour, pumpkin pie spice, and salt. Mix the ingredients well.
4. In another bowl, mix mashed banana, pumpkin puree, vanilla extract and maple syrup. Mix these ingredients well and pour them into the other bowl containing dry ingredients.
5. Add coconut oil and mix well to incorporate it with the mixture.

1.

2. Add chocolate chips and fold them in the batter.
3. Scoop out a tablespoonful of batter on the baking sheet for each cookie. Make as many cookies as needed to finish the batter.
4. Sprinkle pumpkin pie spice on top of the cookies.
5. Put the baking sheet in the oven and cook for 25-30 minutes. The cookies will become golden brown.
6. Take the baking sheet out of the oven and let cool.
7. Serve after cooling them.
8. You can store the remaining cookies in the refrigerator in an airtight jar.

METHOD (for cream filling):

1. Put all the ingredients of cream filling into a medium sized bowl, and stir well to combine.
2. Make ice-cream in the ice-cream maker.

ASSEMBLING THE COOKIES:

1. Place a few cookies upside down and put a scoop of cream filling in the center. Top it with another cookie with its bottom facing the cream.
2. Refrigerate for a while and serve. The ice-cream should be placed in the cookies sandwiches while they are still warm. It makes it easy to assemble the cookies.

Conclusion

We hope that you have enjoyed the delicious cookies and desserts in *Gluten Free Paleo Cookies*. You might never have realized that cookies and brownies can be made in so many different ways. There are many options to explore new things with limited ingredients. You do not have to indulge in unhealthy things to savor the taste of some of the best foods in the world.

You can also take your Paleo diet to another level. Host a Paleo party at your place, and tell your friends to come prepared for cooking as well as eating healthy. It is so much fun eating food that you have cooked together with friends. And, this is not just a girls' thing to indulge in; you can call in the guys as well! They should also know about this concept of eating healthily. Convince them to leave the comfort of their beds and come to your place for cooking on a weekend. We are sure that you will all have fun together.

You can also make suitable changes to the recipes mentioned in this book. Just evaluate the changes your additional ingredients will make to the basic recipe. Alternatively, you can substitute one component with another. A small change in a recipe can make a huge difference. But obviously, the change should be positive. You would not like to eat a cookie as hard as stone! Be cautious while baking and the result will definitely be positive. Go ahead and enjoy the treat of cookies and desserts, guilt-free!